The Origin of Amyotrophic Lateral Sclerosis - Insights into mitochondrial uncoupling and cellular starvation
Hoffmann, Michael

ABOUT THE AUTHOR

Dr. Michael Hoffmann was born in 1973 in Düsseldorf, the capital city of North-Rhine-Westphalia in Germany. He studied biology and finished his Doctoral Thesis in 2004 at the Institute of Genetics, Heinrich-Heine University, Düsseldorf. For one year he taught students of medicine and pharmacy in biochemistry at the Friedrich-Wilhelms-University in Bonn. After another year as postdoc in the department of general pediatrics, he started his own projects on mitochondrial function and aging until 2013. He founded the Institute für Wissenschaftliche Medizin in 2014 and is currently working on the theory for initiation of Amyotrophic Lateral Sclerosis (ALS). Dr. Michael Hoffmann is an expert in molecular biology, genetics, developmental biology and mitochondrial function.

Selected Publications

Hoffmann M, Bellance N, Rossignol R, Koopman W, Willems P, Mayatepek E, Bossinger O, Distelmaier F. *C. elegans ATAD-3 Is Essential for Mitochondrial Activity and Development.* PLoS One (2009). PMID: 19888333

Hoffmann M, Segbert C, Helbig, G, Bossinger O. *Intestinal tube formation in Caenorhabditis elegans requires vang-1 and egl-15 signaling.* Dev. Biol. (2010). PMID: 2000418

Hoffmann M, Honnen S, Mayatepek E, Wätjen W, Bossinger O, Distelmaier F. *MICS-1 interacts with mitochondrial ATAD-3 and modulates lifespan in C. elegans.* Exp. Geront. (2012). PMID: 22245785

Hoffmann M. *Enhanced Uncoupling of the Mitochondrial Respiratory Chain as a Potential Source for Amyotrophic Lateral Sclerosis.* Front. Neurol. (2013). doi: 10.3389/fneur.2013.00086

Hoffmann M. *Vicious Circle of Metaboreflex Dysregulation in Amyotrophic Lateral Sclerosis.* AASCIT communications (2014).

The Origin of Amyotrophic Lateral Sclerosis - Insights into mitochondrial uncoupling and cellular starvation

Hoffmann, Michael

SUMMARY

Each living cell requires energy in form of ATP for most of its processes. This energy is provided within a cell in a compartment that is termed mitochondrion. Within mitochondria, action of the mitochondrial respiratory chain generates the energy using electrons and oxygen. However and because the mitochondrial respiratory chain is so powerful, a side product of ATP is harmful ROS. During physical exercise energy demand increases, which is covered by a raised activity of the mitochondrial respiratory chain. But consequently, the risk of cellular damage inflicted by ROS also increases. To avoid damage done to cellular components, healthy individuals hold capable defense systems against ROS, notably enzymes of the GST, SOD and UCP classes.

Of these, the UCP system is particularly noteworthy because of its capability to operate before ROS is generated. This UCP function is achieved by a reduction of the proton gradient across the inner mitochondrial membrane.

However, because the proton gradient is coupled to ATP generation, a reduction of this gradient consequently diminishes energy production. This means that a cell has to deliberate whether ROS should be prevented at the cost of its cellular energy levels.

But what happens if UCP activity is induced by external events or by exposure to specific substances that evoke a permanent energy deficit? In this book the physiological consequences of enhanced UCP activity are explained and as a result, can be connected to the origin of the neurodegenerative disease amyotrophic lateral sclerosis. Thus, potential treatment opportunities are provided that are missing so far. Further in this context, known risk factors for the initiation of ALS are discussed.

Abbreviations: ALS (Amyotrophic Lateral Sclerosis), ATP (Adenosine Triphosphate), GST (Glutathione S-Transferase), ROS (Reactive Oxygen Species), SOD (Superoxide Dismutase), UCP (Uncoupling Protein)

The cover picture of this book shows the mitochondrial network of a muscle cell in a transgenic model organism, visualized by fluorescence protein and captured on a convokal laser microscope.

The Origin of Amyotrophic Lateral Sclerosis - Insights into mitochondrial uncoupling and cellular starvation

Hoffmann, Michael

INTRODUCTION

Energy generation is the most fundamental task within cells. Mitochondria are essential to maintain both the steady state of energy levels within a cell as well as counteract the risk of energy deficits in times of an increased ATP consumption, especially in muscle cells during physical exercise.

To fulfill this important task, mitochondria are capable to raise ATP production by enhancing the proton gradient across the inner mitochondrial membrane. Because ATP production at complex V of the respiratory chain requires protons that drive the ATP-Synthase, energy production is coupled to the proton gradient.

Consequently, if the proton gradient is reduced, energy production is in turn diminished. On the other hand as a side effect of an enhanced proton gradient and raised energy production, ROS formation increases. It is believed, that retrograde migration of electrons back to complex I of the respiratory chain is the main cause of ROS formation during conditions of high energy demand.

A set of potent defense mechanisms exists to counteract harmful ROS, example given enzymes of GST and SOD classes. Also, enzymes of the UCP class anticipate ROS generation by effectively reducing the proton gradient.

Because of their outstanding role in regulation of as well ATP and ROS generation, UCP class proteins are the main topic and are discussed in more detail. This book is subdivided into the following chapters:

Chapter I) Regulation of mitochondrial respiratory chain activity - What are uncoupling proteins?

Chapter II) Regulation of uncoupling protein activity - Unleash Pandora´s Box.

Chapter III) Cellular starvation and combined exposure as ALS initiators.

Chapter IV) How to potentially avoid ALS and who should be cautious.

The Origin of Amyotrophic Lateral Sclerosis - Insights into mitochondrial uncoupling and cellular starvation
Hoffmann, Michael

Chapter I) Regulation of mitochondrial respiratory chain activity - What are uncoupling proteins?

To understand the origin of amyotrophic lateral sclerosis it is important to know, that energy demand of a cell is covered by action of the so called mitochondrial respiratory chain (MRC).

Mitochondria are the main source for ATP, which is an essential energy carrier required for the majority of cellular processes. It has to be noted, that ATP generated within the mitochondrial network of a cell is mostly used for self-sustaining processes.

However, ATP can be released to the extracellular milieu and is recognized by purinergic receptors at the cell surface to regulate a broad spectrum of responses (1).

The main purpose of the MRC is to generate ATP. Electrons from reduction equivalents NADH and $FADH_2$, deriving from catabolic pathways, are introduced to be transmitted to oxygen. The efficiency of ATP production can be altered by demand, by certain drugs or by pathological processes.

The MRC locates at the inner mitochondrial membrane and is typically separated into five complexes. Introduced electrons at complexes I or II migrate through the complexes III and IV and are finally transmitted to molecular oxygen at complex V.

Oxygen is supplied by the blood stream to the organs and tissues, and enters a cell by diffusion. Without oxygen as the final electron acceptor no ATP can be produced (see **fig. 1**). In each mitochondrion a great number of complexes I-V are present, and mitochondria are typically organized into networks.

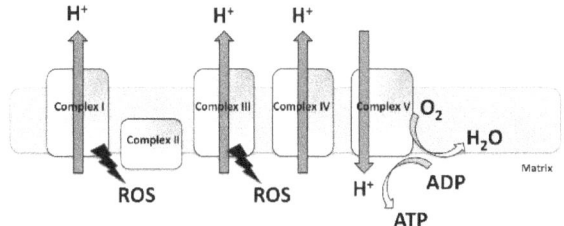

Figure 1: Working principle of the mitochondrial respiratory chain.
Five multi protein complexes localize at the inner mitochondrial membrane and contribute to generation of energy which is needed for most cellular processes. To generate ATP, the mitochondrial respiratory chain essentially requires electrons, that are introduced at complexes I or II, oxygen at complex V as final acceptor for the electrons and the proton gradient. A side product of energy generation is harmful ROS, which can originate at complex I or III.

Chemical energy is generated during the migration of the electrons on their way through the MRC, which is directly used to establish a proton gradient across the inner mitochondrial membrane by exporting proton ions out of the mitochondrial matrix at complexes I, III and IV.

At complex V, which is also termed ATP-Synthase, the proton gradient is necessary to actuate the enzymatic reaction which allows ATP generation deriving from the energy transfer of electrons to oxygen.

Electrons itself are highly reactive particles, thus on their migration through the MRC are always linked to specific transporter proteins, e.g. ubichinone or cytochromes. Reactions of electrons to any other molecules can occur, because in rare cases these electrons escape from their carrier proteins during transfer processes.

This is associated with the activity of complexes I and III. Hereby, reactive oxygen species (ROS) and its progenitors/intermediates can emerge, which what the name already suggests are likewise highly reactive and harmful particles, that on contact are capable to damage any cellular components (2).

Mitochondria can produce a large part of the total ROS made in cells. Formation of ROS under physiological circumstances is kept within narrow borders and is restricted by various very potent defense mechanisms.

For instance, antioxidants like certain vitamins or flavonoids are able to present a reactive double bond which can directly eliminate ROS (3).

Furthermore, specific enzymes are specialized to disarm ROS before damage could be inflicted. The most important proteins to perform this task are enzymes of the classes SOD and GST.

Both systems work very efficiently, but are in need of recharge because they interact directly with the progenitor of ROS. SOD enzymes are metalloproteins and catalyze the dismutation of radicals to uncharged and less harmful molecules by adding or removing electrons (2).

GSTs catalyze the conjugation of the reduced form of glutathione (GSH) to harmful substrates for the purpose of detoxification (4). However, one might think about that the most efficient defense against any harmful action might be just to prevent its origin.

The advantage would be that there is no direct interaction with ROS or its progenitors, hence no need of a recharge and also no exhaustion. And indeed, enzymes of the UCP class possess this special ability to indirectly counteract ROS before it is generated.

Such enzymes, although not characterized into very detail so far, are called uncoupling proteins (UCPs) (5). UCPs manage to control ROS formation before it occurs. UCPs are capable to diminish the proton gradient to such an extend, that ROS formation can be dramatically reduced.

Which signaling pathways control activity of UCPs within a cell is not known yet. However, a tight interplay between other ROS fighting systems exists. In case GST/GSH system or SOD enzymes reach their capacity to fight ROS, a feedback that activates UCP enzymes for cellular protection is enabled (6, 7).

By activation of UCPs the mitochondrial network is capable to adjust the MRC activity under certain conditions, e.g. during physical exercise or exposure to a cold environment.

Direct result of uncoupling activity is that the proton gradient is diminished, which in turn reduces ROS formation but also disables ATP production.

It has been demonstrated, that during physical exercise UCP activity in skeletal muscle raises (8). At the first glance it seems to be conflictive to reduce the proton gradient and the coupled ATP synthesis during physical exercise, a situation in which an enhanced demand of ATP exist.

However it seems to be crucial, that in times of an elevated MRC activity the formation of ROS is limited by uncoupling. For example if oxygen levels are low but the proton gradient is enhanced, sufficient acceptors for electrons are missing.

Here, uncoupling reduces the elevated risk of ROS formation due to backward migration of electrons, even if this situation would last for a couple of seconds only.

Also, if ADP levels are low but oxygen levels are high, uncoupling must reduce the proton gradient which otherwise lead to backward migration of electrons to complex I that results in enhanced ROS formation.

However, to which extend and within which range certain UCPs are capable to adjust ATP production during specific conditions has not been studied in detail so far.

Nevertheless, measurement of ATP production and comparison studies of the proton gradient, indirectly visualized by mitochondrial uptake of cationic staining dyes, suggest options between mild forms of uncoupling as well as very strong uncoupling activity (9, 10).

As a result of uncoupling, potential energy carried by the electrons that migrate through the respiratory chain is set free as heat, which controls body temperature maintenance of homeothermic organisms regulated by brown adipose tissue (BAT) and skeletal muscles (11).

As a side effect of physical exercise as well as uncoupling, the pH value in skeletal muscles is altered which supports activity of the muscle sympathetic nerve (MSNA) (12).

Modulated MSNA directly effects and maintains oxygen supply to the muscle cells which are in need because of enhanced MRC activity and requirement of oxygen as electron acceptor.

Thus, uncoupling activity during physical exercise one the one hand reduce ATP production, but on the other hand also ensures supply of oxygen that is required for ongoing respiratory chain activity, either to generate heat or ATP (see **fig.2**).

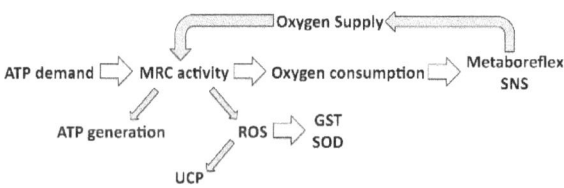

Figure 2: Systemic response on ATP demand includes oxygen supply to ensure MRC activity.
For the mitochondrial respiratory chain (MRC) to work, oxygen as the final electron acceptor is required. To provide proper amounts of oxygen to muscle cells during physical exercise, the metaboreflex activates the sympathetic nervous system (SNS). Oxygen delivery not only ensures MRC activity, but also enhances ROS production.

Hence, uncouplers play an important role in thermoregulation, especially if an organism is exposed to a cold environment and consequently has to counteract for maintenance of its body temperature. In mammals and remarkably as well in plants, uncoupling proteins are induced by cold (13, 14).

In mammals, BAT actively produces heat by mitochondrial uncoupling, which is triggered by thyroid hormone and the sympathetic nervous system (15, 16). It has been proposed, that in human adults uncouplers in skeletal muscles additionally play a role in thermogenesis (11).

In case a cell is stimulated to uncouple the MRC, energy production is consequently reduced. Because MRC activity is the main source for cellular energy, substitutions are always less effective however necessary to avoid short term energy deficits.

Fatty acids are valuable alternative energy carriers if uncoupling is raised but energy demand exists. Nevertheless it is not known to which extend fatty acids can substitute a reduced respiratory chain ATP production in times of enhanced uncoupling activity.

It is also not known, which role is designated to creatine, an energy carrier that can be used by muscle cells and neurons. Further, in non-degenerated cells supply of glucose for ATP production via glycolysis is possible in short terms and could counteract this energy deficit fractional only.

In particular, motoneurons are highly sensitive against a reduction of ATP production and in this regard it has been already demonstrated, that motoneurons rapidly die if the MRC is uncoupled (17, 18).

ATP is not only an energy carrier, it is also necessary to synthesize cyclic adenosine monophosphate (cAMP), which is a second messenger and an important signaling molecule.

If the ATP level in a cell declines because of enhanced uncoupling activity, effects on cAMP signaling might consequently occur. In this regard, activity of Protein kinase A (PKA), a target of cAMP pathway, which regulates glycogen metabolism could be modulated. Thus, the immediate energy reserve glycogen, which is controlled by PKA, may not be available to muscle cells that exhibit an increased UCP activity.

Because of difficulties in experimental set up to directly verify uncoupling in living cells, it is problematic to identify uncoupling activity of a protein.

Indirect data that support uncoupling activity derive from evidences found by visualizing the proton gradient at the inner mitochondrial membrane by cationic staining dyes, e.g. tetramethylrhodamine methyl ester (TMRM) *in vivo* (19, 20).

Also a localization at MRC complexes should exist for a candidate protein to function as an uncoupler (16). In addition, diminishing of ROS formation by uncoupling activity should be measurable (21).

Despite the fact that fundamental *in vivo* studies about UCPs function and regulation are missing, five uncoupling proteins have been identified in human so far

(14). They are designated as UCP1-UCP5, and display moderate sequence homology among one another which suggests different mechanisms of proton gradient reduction, respectively.

Thus, the exact nature of UCPs as well as their site of interaction has not been fully described yet and is subject to ongoing research. Example given, UCPs may be involved in the handling of lipids, demonstrating the complex interaction of energy generation and ROS regulation at the respiratory chain (22).

Systemic and anatomic expression profiles of UCPs are dynamic and complex, supporting the importance of uncoupling activity contributing to regulation of the MRC.

Different UCPs are active during development of an organism. Furthermore, a tissue specificity for UCPs seem to exist (23, 24). Also, sex dependent regulation of UCP activity has been demonstrated (25).

All UCPs have in common, that they are encoded by nuclear DNA and locate to the inner mitochondrial membrane (26). UCP1-UCP5 are members of the mitochondrial anion carrier protein family. UCP1 shares 59% and 57% sequence homology with UCP2 and UCP3, respectively (27).

UCP1 expression initially was found to be restricted to BAT, presumably due to its important role in thermoregulation, whereas UCP2 is widely expressed including adipose tissue, muscle, lymphocytes, heart and brain (28, 29). UCP2 is also highly conserved among species, displaying 95% homology between human and murine sequences.

The amino acid sequence of UCP3 is 57% identical to that of UCP1 and 73% identical to that of UCP2. UCP3 is expressed in skeletal muscle, BAT and in the heart and expression of UCP1-3 has also been found in human keratinocytes (27, 30).

UCP4 is expressed in brain, adipose tissues and skeletal muscle (31). UCP5 is predominantly expressed in neural tissues (32).

UCP activity to limit ROS formation under physiological conditions is not restricted to the tissues mentioned above, but can also be found in the immune system. Macrophages for example use ROS to fight encounters, and UCP2 mutant mice are more resistant to *Toxoplasma* infections due to enhanced formation of ROS in their macrophages (33).

Using environmental oxygen for energy generation was a milestone in evolution. However, the opportunity to generate vast amounts of ATP bears the raised risk of cellular damage inflicted by ROS.

Thus, defense mechanisms evolved that are capable to disarm ROS but also to completely avoid ROS generation at the expense of ATP production. Regulation of the cellular defense machinery that fight ROS is not completely understood, nevertheless misregulation of uncoupling activity might induce an energy deficit that contributes to the etiology of motor neuron diseases.

The Origin of Amyotrophic Lateral Sclerosis - Insights into mitochondrial uncoupling and cellular starvation
Hoffmann, Michael

Chapter II) Regulation of uncoupling protein activity - Unleash Pandora´s Box.

Mitochondrial uncoupling reduces ROS formation as well as ATP production. In addition to uncoupling activation by exposure to cold environment or by physical exercise, a number of conditions have been described that are capable to induce uncoupling as well.

Notably, cellular stress can modulate mitochondrial uncoupling as part of stress response mechanism. For instance, certain toxic substances are capacitated to enhance ROS levels within a cell (2). In such a case, uncoupling is activated to support the ROS defense machinery and to avoid possible damage inflicted by ROS.

Enzymes of the SOD and GST classes shape the mainstay of cellular stress response. One disadvantage of SOD and GST enzymes might be, that the activity of these enzymes depends in principle on entire redox state within a cell.

Hence, both systems can be dismantled by an increased reaction of their catalytic center to electrons, which can occur e.g. during continuous exercise or by exposure to heavy metals or toxic substances, without having the time to recharge.

That might be one of the reasons why UCPs are directly activated in situations of elevated ROS formation, because UCP activity can not be stopped by redox reactions.

"The cellular ATP level acts likewise a battery for UCP activity to ensure ROS repression."

If SOD and GST defense capabilities are lowered by raised ROS occurrence, UCPs remain active at the expense of ATP production. If in any situation SOD and GST however can fight ROS, UCPs activity is diminished which in turn restores ATP levels (see **fig. 3**).

In theory, UCPs possess an unlimited capacity to disable ROS formation at the MRC as long as sufficient amounts of ATP can be generated or are present to also cover cellular energy demand. Thus, the cellular ATP level acts likewise a battery for UCP activity to ensure ROS repression.

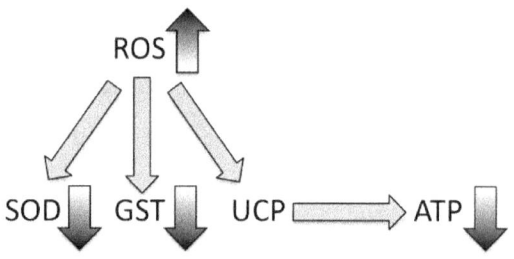

Figure 3: Sustaining ROS reduces SOD and GST defense but not UCP.
SOD and GST activity depend in principle on their capability to "catch electrons". This action requires time to recharge. If ROS is permanently generated, SOD and GST activity decline. The MRC is the major source of ROS within a cell. UCPs act directly on the MRC by removing the proton motif force, which can diminish ROS generation. However, ATP production is also affected by UCP activity. Thus, a cell literally has to choose between starvation (i.e. reduced ATP production) or raised risk of cellular damage in times of enhanced ROS formation.

Variable mutations in respective genes, which reduce the operational readiness of SOD or GST enzymes, have been described in certain types of neurodegenerative diseases.

In this regard, sensitivity of SOD mutant mice to cellular stress is displayed by the development of a phenotype that resembles amyotrophic lateral sclerosis (ALS), a disease that is mainly characterized by muscle wasting and degeneration of motoneurons (34).

Cumulative mutations that alter SOD activity have been isolated in humans which exhibit familiar ALS (35, 36). Hence, a diminished capacity in fighting ROS under certain circumstances seem to participate in the pathogenesis of some ALS forms.

> A fundamental principle states that prevention of ROS by UCP activity is more important than creating an energy deficit by the same action.

Noteworthy in this context, if SOD or GSH activity is diminished, UCP activity consequently raises to substitute deficits in

27

stress response and to counteract ROS formation. With enhanced UCP activity the capability of the respiratory chain to generate ATP declines.

Thus, a fundamental principle states that prevention of ROS by UCP activity is more important than creating an energy deficit by the same action.

To date, several substances have been described to induce mitochondrial uncoupling. To which extend any one-time or chronic exposure of organisms to such substances is harmful is difficult to track and remains to be shown in detail (37).

However, most of the substances that can trigger mitochondrial uncoupling have also been suggested to function as potential candidates for the initiation of ALS.

Notably in connection with this, heavy metals like selenium (38, 39), mercury (40, 41) or cadmium (42, 43) have been demonstrated to uncouple mitochondria as well as have been classified as risk factors for ALS initiation.

Other chemical compounds like 2,4-dinitrophenole (DNP) or carbonyl-cyanide-p-trifluoromethoxyphenylhydrazone (FCCP) are uncoupling agents as well.

Detailed studies on DNP or FCCP with respect to its impact on ALS development are missing so far, however it has been noticed that certain population subgroups display a raised ALS incidence which might be connected to the prolonged or repeated ingestion of DNP.

DNP can be used to metaphorically speaking burn body fat and therefore shape the body for esthetical reasons, which is commonly performed by active or professional body builders (44).

DNP intake contributes to an energy deficit by enhanced uncoupling of the MRC, which is compensated by body fat reserves to cover energy demand (45, 46). Thus, it seems possible to encounter the energy deficits generated by mitochondrial uncoupling by using fatty acids to an undefined extend.

On the other hand it also seems likely that if body fat reserves are low, capabilities to face energy deficits due to enhanced or maintained uncoupling without developing ALS are limited.

In this context it has to be mentioned, that people developing ALS are slim and versatile if compared to control groups (47). ALS incidence in body builders seem to be raised, however specific and detailed information on DNP administration are missing which leaves open any opportunity to classify the impact of DNP on ALS initiation.

It has been shown that application of FCCP in healthy subjects uncouples the respiratory chain and enhances oxygen consumption.

However, in ALS patients FCCP misses enhancement of oxygen consumption (48). An explanation of this phenomenon would be that in ALS patients mitochondrial uncoupling is already enhanced and has reached a physiological limit to such an extend, that any further attempt to induce uncoupling by FCCP remains without effect.

In fact it has been demonstrated that in ALS model systems as well as in ALS patients UCP activity is raised and uncoupling activity contributes to accelerated ALS progression (19, 49, 50).

Modulation of MRC activity by uncoupling proteins can also be induced by physiological intrinsic elicitors.

To start with the spatially closest encounter, overproduction of ROS by the MRC itself activates uncoupling to diminish forthcoming ROS formation (51).

Further, 4-hydroxynonenal (4-HNE) is an unsaturated aldehyde and a product of lipid oxidation, and also capable to activate uncoupling. 4-HNE indirectly increases ROS by reacting with glutathione, thereby depleting cells of this critical component of the stress defense system (52, 53).

Whether it is feasible to extrapolate induction of lipid oxidation by energy deficits, thus reducing GST/GSH system, to a consequently raised uncoupling activity which finally leads to enhanced risk of ALS in the above mentioned context remains to be shown (26, 54).

It is noteworthy, however, that in ALS patients 4-HNE is significantly increased (51, 55). This observation might suggest that enhanced uncoupling evokes an energy deficit which in attempt for compensation activates alternative energy sources (34).

Catecholamines, retinoids and thyroid hormones greatly activate expression of UCPs in various tissues, whereas administration of corticosterone lowers UCP levels (14).

The regulation by thyroid hormones emphasizes the important contribution of uncoupling proteins to the physiology and metabolism of the whole organism.

Indeed it has been shown, that enhanced uncoupling activity in skeletal muscle influences the systemic metabolism, altering oxygen supply and glucose uptake (56).

Biochemical data on UCP inhibition demonstrate an even more complex regulation of UCP activity. In this regard, GDP and ADP as well as GTP and ATP are capable to inhibit UCPs (57). Thus it remains to be determined, which energy sensor or signaling pathway is capable to identify cellular ATP levels and deficits, and consequently regulates the activity of UCPs (3).

Given the paradigm for mitochondria, that fighting ROS is the most important task even outweigh energy generation by the MRC, a vicious circle is revealed (58).

The critical point is, that UCP malfunction removes ATP generation, but the physiological effects to cover ATP demand remain active (see **fig. 4**).

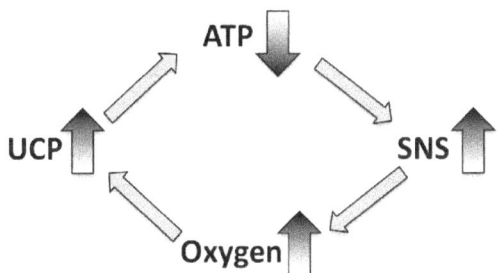

Figure 4: Vicious Circle evoked by maintained UCP activity.
UCP activity reduces the cellular ATP level. This is recognized by mechanisms which activate the SNS to deliver oxygen. However, oxygen can not be used and promotes continuous UCP activity.

In particular, the SNS acts to compensate for UCP induced energy deficits by enhancing oxygen supply via the blood flow.

As stated above, oxygen is necessary for the MRC to accept the electrons and drive ATP generation at complex V. However, because UCP activity removes the proton motif force, no ATP can be generated by the MRC but electrons are still introduced and transferred to oxygen.

In turn, UCPs must remain active due to the high risk of ROS formation based upon both electron flow and presence of oxygen.

The Origin of Amyotrophic Lateral Sclerosis - Insights into mitochondrial uncoupling and cellular starvation
Hoffmann, Michael

Chapter III) Cellular starvation and combined exposure as ALS initiators.

A human body is able to survive in the absence of nutrition. After prolonged periods of low energy intake, a particular symptom of starvation is skeletal muscle wasting. Glucogenic amino acids from skeletal muscles are used for gluconeogenesis to provide glucose and to support energy for the brain, hence leading to muscle mass degradation. In this context, a principle of homeostasis describes the brain giving priority to regulating its own ATP concentrations by allocation of energy from the periphery (59).

"A principle of homeostasis describes the brain giving priority to regulating its own ATP concentrations by allocation of energy from the periphery."

Because skeletal muscle wasting is a symptom of ALS, one might ask whether it is possible to establish a direct connection between ALS and the physiological response to starvation.

In this regard the question arises, whether an energy deficit induced by maintained uncoupling protein activity in skeletal muscles is sufficient to be interpreted as a period of cellular starvation. In the course of a physiological response, the brain incorrectly starts to protect itself by application of ATP priority.

Unfortunately, mechanisms that recognize starvation and regulate energy fluxes in the organism are not understood to such an extend which would definitively allow the combination of cellular starvation to the origin of ALS yet.

Nevertheless, by focusing on stress response and cellular energy deficits triggered by UCPs, cellular starvation and its systemic response may contribute to the development of ALS.

Muscle cramps in early stage of ALS, for example, could therefore be a direct symptom of ATP deficiency, and may not primarily be a sign of motoneuron malfunction.

Remarkably, thyroid dysfunction was investigated for centuries specifically with regard to ALS initiation. Thyroid hormones are responsible for regulation of metabolism, they increase the basal metabolic rate and also regulate heat generation.

In this context, thyroid hyperfunction is one established differential diagnosis to ALS, mimicking pathological nervous system alterations and notably muscle wasting (60).

As stated above, thyroid hormones are also known to activate UCPs (11, 61). Hence, muscle wasting in hyperthyroidism could based upon enhanced UCP activity, which diminishes the cellular ATP level. Consequently, the physiological responses which lead to muscle wasting in hyperthyroidism are comparably to the responses in ALS, and both conditions originate in enhanced UCP activity.

Further support for the hypothesis of cellular starvation derives from a very different disease. To imagine that cellular starvation *per se* could be triggered by different events, other conditions presenting with skeletal muscle wasting must exist.

Indeed, skeletal muscle wasting is also a symptom in chronic heart failure. In this disease, increased ROS play an important role in skeletal muscle wasting during physical exercise (62).

Of note, failing hearts have increased UCP expression (63). On the one hand, UCPs are necessary to counteract the risk of ROS formation. But on the other hand, ATP levels decline if UCPs are active.

It is not known how this information regarding cellular energy deficits is recognized by the central nervous system, but sensitization of the metaboreflex might play an important role (64).

It is striking that physical exercise is frequently connected to the development of ALS. It is also striking that skeletal muscle wasting is virtually the opposite of what would be achieved by physical exercise.

It seems that in periods of high energy demand, specifically during exercise, initiation of ALS is more likely. Not only because UCP activity is raised during physical exercise, the connection of an energy deficit and ALS development is feasible (see **fig. 5**).

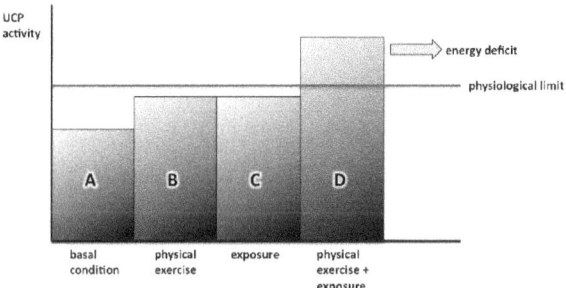

Figure 5: UCP activity can exceed a physiological limit.
(A) In a normal state, UCPs are active because of their important contribution to stress response and thermoregulation. (B) During physical exercise, UCP activity is shifted. (C) Also, exposure to herbicides, electricity or heavy metals increases UCP activity. (D) After contact and if a person performs physical exercise, the physiological limit is exceeded.

A basal UCP activity would never pass the physiological limit, which would allow onset of ALS due to an energy deficiency, because it is tightly regulated.

Even physical activity alone can not be sufficient to pass this limit. However, interference with regulatory mechanisms either by enhancing UCP activity directly or indirectly by dismantling SOD or GST/GSH systems in combination with physical activity seems to exceed the physiological limit.

Diversified studies that fit inside this theory of combined UCP misregulation can be found by the observed enhanced ALS incidence, e.g. in agricultural workers, soccer players, bodybuilders or people exposed to heavy metals (43, 44, 65-68).

The increased ALS incidence in these groups would be explainable by combination of physical exercise or heavy physical labor and exposure to uncoupling agents like herbicides, DNP or heavy metals, respectively.

As a conclusion it seems likely that more than one misregulation of uncoupling must exist, e.g. thyroid hormone imbalance or enhanced lipid oxidation in combination with exposure to heavy metals, herbicides or electricity (see **fig. 6**). It has been suggested that enhanced ALS incidence in professional Italian soccer players might be due to contact with herbicides, a finding that could support the combined exposure theory, in this regard physical exercise and exposure to herbicides (69).

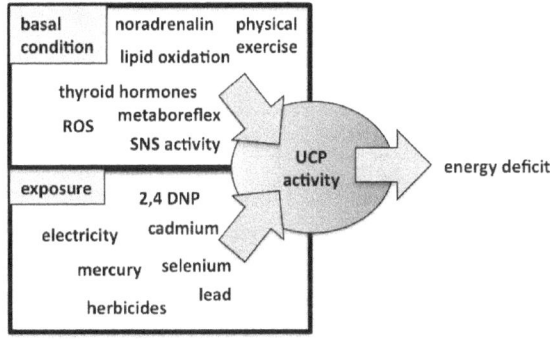

Figure 6: Combined influences on UCP activity can cause the pathological energy deficit.

The raised incidence of ALS in certain population subgroups is explainable by a sustaining energy deficit, induced either by chronic exposure or even a single contact to the substances enlisted in the lower part of the figure. In combination with e.g. physical exercise or enhanced lipid oxidation, UCP activity exceeds the physiological limit that creates an energy deficit.

It might be worth to mention at this point, that besides the direct contact at work, exposure to toxic substances in urban regions is likewise higher than in more rural regions. In combination with current lifestyle activities, in particular performing sports after work, the risk of increasing the ALS incidence in urban regions is given.

"The risk of increasing ALS incidence in urban regions is given."

To date only a few substances which are capable to block UCP activity are known. Genipin is such a substance, that has already been tested to inhibit uncoupling activity in isolated pancreatic islets to reverse beta cell dysfunction (70). Genipin is a geniposide and a component of gardenia fructus which is used in traditional Asian herbal medicine (71). To the authors knowledge, impact of Genipin application on ALS progression has not been studied so far.

Further, ginseng extracts include unknown substances that are also capable to inhibit uncouplers (72). Remarkably in this context, although the number of subjects was limited, a study already describes the possibility to slow down ALS progression by application of ginseng extracts (73).

Identification of novel substances that are capable to block UCP activity would be relatively simple. Easy to handle model organisms like *C. elegans* or *D. melanogaster* provide powerful molecular biology tools to study the effects of diverse substances on UCP activity.

Specifically *C. elegans* is already utilized in screens covering diverse aspects, and administration of substances is generally well. Even experiments on cell culture should be sufficient to test effects of potential UCP inhibitors easily.

It would be interesting to elucidate whether measurements of UCP activity or antibody testing of human blood samples could be used as diagnostic tools to predict individual ALS onset and progression, comparably to creatine kinase (CK) value determination.

However it is not known so far, whether UCPs in the course of muscle wasting are released into the bloodstream. Ever since ALS is known for over 100 years, no treatment has been established. Understanding of so far unknown physiological responses to cellular starvation seems to be crucial to counteract energy deficits generated by enhanced uncoupling of the MRC.

The Origin of Amyotrophic Lateral Sclerosis - Insights into mitochondrial uncoupling and cellular starvation
Hoffmann, Michael

Chapter IV) How to potentially avoid ALS and who should be cautious.

Analysis of the data on professional soccer players died from ALS revealed that after exposure to herbicides and start of physical exercise, a mean time span of about 17-19 years passed until ALS developed (69).

In between, most of the players already quit their professional sports career, and no correlation exists in how long soccer was played. Which means, it is not crucial how long or intense an exposure to herbicides must have taken place to develop ALS.

This is an interesting finding, because one conclusion is that ALS requires an initiation event to disrupt energy homeostasis. It seems that once mitochondria are manipulated, malfunction slowly spreads and can not be repaired.

However, because not the majority from the respective soccer teams developed ALS, either protective mechanisms are individually different or a repair is still possible. In context of the vicious circle mentioned above, individual capabilities to face cellular energy deficits seems to be more likely.

In sports, electrotherapy to support healing processes is not uncommon, and professional football players in the US display a higher ALS incidence (66).

Exposure to electromagnetic fields and electricity is associated with an increased risk to develop ALS, which has been analyzed in a study on men employed in utility companies in Denmark (74).

The apparent causal relation between working in electrical jobs and development of ALS is supported by similar observations made in Sweden and in the US. In this context it has been shown that electricity enhances UCP activity (75).

The time span between first employment and death for most subjects is

10-29 years, however the time point of exposure to electric shocks in accidents is documented in one case only. Here, an electric shock occurred 19 years prior to the diagnosis of ALS.

This truly might be coincidence, but is in the range of ALS initiation of soccer players exposed to herbicides. Given the fact that accidents and consequent exposure to electricity is a random event, the time span to develop ALS because of electricity might be much shorter.

Contact to heavy metals like selenium or cadmium is a common cause for ALS. Heavy metals strongly uncouple the MRC, either by unknown mechanisms, by their ability to produce ROS or its progenitors and/or by depletion of glutathione. Hence, ALS initiation subsequent to heavy metal exposure seems to be faster than after electrotherapy. In this context it has been described that 9 years after exposure to cadmium a factory worker died from ALS (43).

It may be assumed that the exposure to ALS initiators is limited to hands or legs in the majority of cases. But how can induced uncoupling in specific parts of the body leads to ALS?

It is not known whether a maintained malfunction of specific mitochondria is sufficient to develop ALS. But this has to be discussed, because certain aspects fit into the here presented essay. One can imagine, that for example the Opponens Pollicis, a muscle in the hand which is innervated by the median nerve, is exposed to some amounts of herbicides. This exposure induces uncoupling which consequently leads to a decline in energy production, but only in mitochondria of this specific muscle.

In case the affected hand is used e.g. for gardening, the metaboreflex is necessary to provide sufficient amounts of oxygen to muscles by regulating the activity of the SNS. In turn, oxygen delivery is increased through the blood flow, but is not restricted to the hand muscles.

The presence of oxygen enhances introduction of electrons into the MRC to produce ATP. The mitochondria in the Opponens Pollicis, however, are not fully capable to use neither the oxygen nor the electrons for energy production, because the MRC is uncoupled.

This activates the vicious circle (58). If the physiological limit in the Opponens Pollicis is reached and an energy deficit emerges, the metaboreflex is continuously activated to deliver oxygen, which finally leads to muscle wasting due to cellular starvation.

Perpetual delivery of oxygen might cause irritation, because in all other cells the energy demand is not raised. As a consequence, uncoupling is activated in all cells to reduce the risk of ROS formation due to the presence of oxygen and enhanced introduction of electrons into the MRC.

At this point it becomes reasonable, that SOD impaired organisms display a higher affinity to develop ALS. Thus, because the SOD system is affected, UCPs are comparably more sensitive and more active.

This vicious circle may be active for years without causing any visible symptoms until ALS is diagnosed. It may also be active without causing any symptoms in a lifetime, depending on the energy deficit and the individually physiological limit.

Also it may possible that after a period of vicious circle activity, other mechanisms are upregulated to counteract the effects. The existence of ALS should reminds us that there are processes within the human body that we do not understand so far.

However, simultaneous prevention of the vicious circle activity seems to be the key to avoid ALS initiation or to slow down the progression (see **fig. 7**). This may be possible in particular by interference with the activity of UCPs and the SNS. Inhibition of UCPs will consequently restore ATP levels, however, clinical trials on UCP inhibitors Genipin, Ginseng or Gardenia are missing up to now.

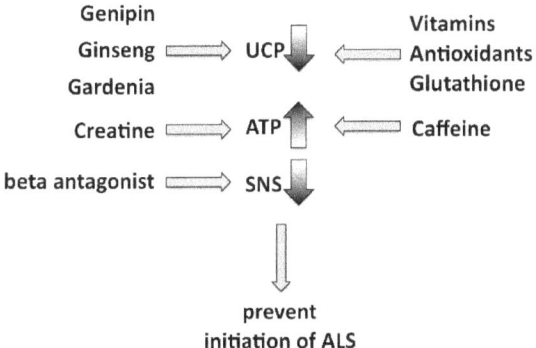

Figure 7: Reduction of UCP and SNS activity and recovery of ATP levels to prevent ALS initiation.

Nevertheless, by supporting the SOD and GST systems, it should be indirectly possible to reduce UCP activity and to restore ATP levels at once. This might be achieved by supplementation with glutathione and with antioxidants to directly react with ROS. In turn, the SOD/GST defense can recharge.

ATP levels, or specifically energy levels, can also be restored by supplementation of creatine to an uncertain

51

extend. ALS patients often report a gain in muscle strength after creatine intake.

It has to be noted that glucose, which is typically a very potent energy carrier, might not be converted to energy efficiently in ALS patients, because the enzyme (i.e. PKA) that is required for proper utilization of glucose is inactivated by the energy deficit that is caused by the vicious circle. PKA activity depends on cAMP level, which based upon short ATP level in ALS.

Caffeine restores levels of the second messenger cAMP and consequently supports activity of the PKA. Hence Caffeine supports accessibility to glucose in ALS. In this regard, an inverse correlation between coffee intake and ALS risk has been documented (76).

Inhibition of SNS and metaboreflex activity is possible by administration of certain drugs, but side effects are common. So called beta-blockers interfere with the function of SNS mediators by blocking signal transduction. It is not known, whether beta-blockers provide a benefit on ALS progression.

In summary, people who have been exposed to electricity, herbicides or heavy metals must take attention not to enhance their risk for developing ALS.

It is important that after contact to ALS initiators, physical exercise should be avoided for weeks. In addition, supplementation of antioxidants and other possible substances to counteract the effects of the vicious circle is important.

It is known, that antioxidants like ascorbic acid, carotonoids or flavonoids are capable of chelating metal ions, reducing their catalytic activity to form ROS.

It is also important to avoid other substances that enhance the metaboreflex or SNS activity, e.g. aspirin. In this context, aspirin has been shown to sensitize the metaboreflex and consequently enhances the progression of ALS (77). We can not heal ALS, thus we have to avoid its formation.

"We can not heal ALS, thus we have to avoid its formation."

REFERENCES

1.   Schwiebert EM, Zsembery A. Extracellular ATP as a signaling molecule for epithelial cells. Biochim Biophys Acta. 2003 Sep 2;1615(1-2):7-32.
2.   Deavall DG, Martin EA, Horner JM, Roberts R. Drug-induced oxidative stress and toxicity. J Toxicol. 2012;2012:645460.
3.   Jezek P, Hlavata L. Mitochondria in homeostasis of reactive oxygen species in cell, tissues, and organism. Int J Biochem Cell Biol. 2005 Dec;37(12):2478-503.
4.   Hayes JD, Pulford DJ. The glutathione S-transferase supergene family: regulation of GST and the contribution of the isoenzymes to cancer chemoprotection and drug resistance. Crit Rev Biochem Mol Biol. 1995;30(6):445-600.
5.   Rousset S, Alves-Guerra MC, Mozo J, Miroux B, Cassard-Doulcier AM, Bouillaud F, et al. The biology of mitochondrial uncoupling proteins. Diabetes. 2004 Feb;53 Suppl 1:S130-5.
6.   de Bilbao F, Arsenijevic D, Vallet P, Hjelle OP, Ottersen OP, Bouras C, et al. Resistance to cerebral ischemic injury in UCP2 knockout mice: evidence for a role of UCP2 as a regulator of mitochondrial glutathione levels. J Neurochem. 2004 Jun;89(5):1283-92.
7.   Pi J, Bai Y, Daniel KW, Liu D, Lyght O, Edelstein D, et al. Persistent oxidative stress due to absence of uncoupling protein 2 associated with impaired pancreatic beta-cell function. Endocrinology. 2009 Jul;150(7):3040-8.
8.   Jiang N, Zhang G, Bo H, Qu J, Ma G, Cao D, et al. Upregulation of uncoupling protein-3 in skeletal muscle during exercise: a potential antioxidant function. Free Radic Biol Med. 2009 Jan 15;46(2):138-45.
9.   Mailloux RJ, Harper ME. Uncoupling proteins and the control of mitochondrial reactive oxygen species production. Free Radic Biol Med. 2011 Sep 15;51(6):1106-15.
10.   Bartolome F, Wu HC, Burchell VS, Preza E, Wray S, Mahoney CJ, et al. Pathogenic VCP Mutations Induce Mitochondrial Uncoupling and Reduced ATP Levels. Neuron. 2013 Mar 13.
11.   Silva JE. Thermogenic mechanisms and their hormonal regulation. Physiol Rev. 2006 Apr;86(2):435-64.
12.   Victor RG, Bertocci LA, Pryor SL, Nunnally RL. Sympathetic nerve discharge is coupled to muscle cell pH during exercise in humans. J Clin Invest. 1988 Oct;82(4):1301-5.

54

13.   Boss O, Samec S, Paoloni-Giacobino A, Rossier C, Dulloo A, Seydoux J, et al. Uncoupling protein-3: a new member of the mitochondrial carrier family with tissue-specific expression. FEBS Lett. 1997 May 12;408(1):39-42.

14.   Ricquier D, Bouillaud F. Mitochondrial uncoupling proteins: from mitochondria to the regulation of energy balance. J Physiol. 2000 Nov 15;529 Pt 1:3-10.

15.   Slocum N, Durrant JR, Bailey D, Yoon L, Jordan H, Barton J, et al. Responses of brown adipose tissue to diet-induced obesity, exercise, dietary restriction and ephedrine treatment. Exp Toxicol Pathol. 2012 Apr 27.

16.   Virtanen KA, Lidell ME, Orava J, Heglind M, Westergren R, Niemi T, et al. Functional brown adipose tissue in healthy adults. N Engl J Med. 2009 Apr 9;360(15):1518-25.

17.   Dupuis L, Gonzalez de Aguilar JL, Echaniz-Laguna A, Eschbach J, Rene F, Oudart H, et al. Muscle mitochondrial uncoupling dismantles neuromuscular junction and triggers distal degeneration of motor neurons. PLoS One. 2009;4(4):e5390.

18.   Kaal EC, Vlug AS, Versleijen MW, Kuilman M, Joosten EA, Bar PR. Chronic mitochondrial inhibition induces selective motoneuron death in vitro: a new model for amyotrophic lateral sclerosis. J Neurochem. 2000 Mar;74(3):1158-65.

19.   Dupuis L, di Scala F, Rene F, de Tapia M, Oudart H, Pradat PF, et al. Up-regulation of mitochondrial uncoupling protein 3 reveals an early muscular metabolic defect in amyotrophic lateral sclerosis. FASEB J. 2003 Nov;17(14):2091-3.

20.   Distelmaier F, Koopman WJ, Testa ER, de Jong AS, Swarts HG, Mayatepek E, et al. Life cell quantification of mitochondrial membrane potential at the single organelle level. Cytometry A. 2008 Feb;73(2):129-38.

21.   Yonezawa T, Kurata R, Hosomichi K, Kono A, Kimura M, Inoko H. Nutritional and hormonal regulation of uncoupling protein 2. IUBMB Life. 2009 Dec;61(12):1123-31.

22.   Weigle DS, Selfridge LE, Schwartz MW, Seeley RJ, Cummings DE, Havel PJ, et al. Elevated free fatty acids induce uncoupling protein 3 expression in muscle: a potential explanation for the effect of fasting. Diabetes. 1998 Feb;47(2):298-302.

23.   Oliver P, Pico C, Palou A. Differential expression of genes for uncoupling proteins 1, 2 and 3 in brown and white adipose tissue depots during rat development. Cell Mol Life Sci. 2001 Mar;58(3):470-6.

24.   Rupprecht A, Brauer AU, Smorodchenko A, Goyn J, Hilse KE, Shabalina IG, et al. Quantification of uncoupling protein

2 reveals its main expression in immune cells and selective up-regulation during T-cell proliferation. PLoS One. 2012;7(8):e41406.

25. Rodriguez AM, Palou A. Uncoupling proteins: gender-dependence and their relation to body weight control. Int J Obes Relat Metab Disord. 2004 Feb;28(2):327-9.

26. Mattiasson G, Sullivan PG. The emerging functions of UCP2 in health, disease, and therapeutics. Antioxid Redox Signal. 2006 Jan-Feb;8(1-2):1-38.

27. Azzu V, Jastroch M, Divakaruni AS, Brand MD. The regulation and turnover of mitochondrial uncoupling proteins. Biochim Biophys Acta. 2010 Jun-Jul;1797(6-7):785-91.

28. Fleury C, Neverova M, Collins S, Raimbault S, Champigny O, Levi-Meyrueis C, et al. Uncoupling protein-2: a novel gene linked to obesity and hyperinsulinemia. Nat Genet. 1997 Mar;15(3):269-72.

29. Gimeno RE, Dembski M, Weng X, Deng N, Shyjan AW, Gimeno CJ, et al. Cloning and characterization of an uncoupling protein homolog: a potential molecular mediator of human thermogenesis. Diabetes. 1997 May;46(5):900-6.

30. Mori S, Yoshizuka N, Takizawa M, Takema Y, Murase T, Tokimitsu I, et al. Expression of uncoupling proteins in human skin and skin-derived cells. J Invest Dermatol. 2008 Aug;128(8):1894-900.

31. Slocinska M, Antos-Krzeminska N, Rosinski G, Jarmuszkiewicz W. Molecular identification and functional characterisation of uncoupling protein 4 in larva and pupa fat body mitochondria from the beetle Zophobas atratus. Comp Biochem Physiol B Biochem Mol Biol. 2012 Aug;162(4):126-33.

32. Sanchis D, Fleury C, Chomiki N, Goubern M, Huang Q, Neverova M, et al. BMCP1, a novel mitochondrial carrier with high expression in the central nervous system of humans and rodents, and respiration uncoupling activity in recombinant yeast. J Biol Chem. 1998 Dec 18;273(51):34611-5.

33. Arsenijevic D, Onuma H, Pecqueur C, Raimbault S, Manning BS, Miroux B, et al. Disruption of the uncoupling protein-2 gene in mice reveals a role in immunity and reactive oxygen species production. Nat Genet. 2000 Dec;26(4):435-9.

34. Wijesekera LC, Leigh PN. Amyotrophic lateral sclerosis. Orphanet J Rare Dis. 2009;4:3.

35. Grieb P. Transgenic models of amyotrophic lateral sclerosis. Folia Neuropathol. 2004;42(4):239-48.

36. Bocci T, Pecori C, Giorli E, Briscese L, Tognazzi S, Caleo M, et al. Differential motor neuron impairment and axonal regeneration in sporadic and familiar amyotrophic lateral

sclerosis with SOD-1 mutations: lessons from neurophysiology. Int J Mol Sci. 2011;12(12):9203-15.

37.   Vinceti M, Guidetti D, Bergomi M, Caselgrandi E, Vivoli R, Olmi M, et al. Lead, cadmium, and selenium in the blood of patients with sporadic amyotrophic lateral sclerosis. Ital J Neurol Sci. 1997 Apr;18(2):87-92.

38.   Kilness AW, Hichberg FH. Amyotrophic lateral sclerosis in a high selenium environment. JAMA. 1977 Jun 27;237(26):2843-4.

39.   Shilo S, Aharoni-Simon M, Tirosh O. Selenium attenuates expression of MnSOD and uncoupling protein 2 in J774.2 macrophages: molecular mechanism for its cell-death and antiinflammatory activity. Antioxid Redox Signal. 2005 Jan-Feb;7(1-2):276-86.

40.   Adams CR, Ziegler DK, Lin JT. Mercury intoxication simulating amyotrophic lateral sclerosis. JAMA. 1983 Aug 5;250(5):642-3.

41.   Konigsberg M, Lopez-Diazguerrero NE, Bucio L, Gutierrez-Ruiz MC. Uncoupling effect of mercuric chloride on mitochondria isolated from an hepatic cell line. J Appl Toxicol. 2001 Jul-Aug;21(4):323-9.

42.   Miccadei S, Floridi A. Sites of inhibition of mitochondrial electron transport by cadmium. Chem Biol Interact. 1993 Dec;89(2-3):159-67.

43.   Bar-Sela S, Reingold S, Richter ED. Amyotrophic lateral sclerosis in a battery-factory worker exposed to cadmium. Int J Occup Environ Health. 2001 Apr-Jun;7(2):109-12.

44.   Manuel M, Heckman CJ. Stronger is not always better: could a bodybuilding dietary supplement lead to ALS? Exp Neurol. 2011 Mar;228(1):5-8.

45.   Witter RF, Newcomb EH, Stotz E. Studies of the mechanism of action of dinitrophenol. J Biol Chem. 1953 May;202(1):291-303.

46.   Sand P, Madsen S. [Dnitrophenol--a dangerous doping agent]. Tidsskr Nor Laegeforen. 2002 May 30;122(14):1363-4.

47.   Chio A, Mora G. Physical fitness and amyotrophic lateral sclerosis: dangerous liaisons or common genetic pathways? J Neurol Neurosurg Psychiatry. 2012 Apr;83(4):389.

48.   Curti D, Malaspina A, Facchetti G, Camana C, Mazzini L, Tosca P, et al. Amyotrophic lateral sclerosis: oxidative energy metabolism and calcium homeostasis in peripheral blood lymphocytes. Neurology. 1996 Oct;47(4):1060-4.

49.   Zhan L, Hanson KA, Kim SH, Tare A, Tibbetts RS. Identification of genetic modifiers of TDP-43 neurotoxicity in Drosophila. PLoS One. 2013;8(2):e57214.

50.   Peixoto PM, Kim HJ, Sider B, Starkov A, Horvath TL, Manfredi G. UCP2 overexpression worsens mitochondrial dysfunction and accelerates disease progression in a mouse model of amyotrophic lateral sclerosis. Mol Cell Neurosci. 2013 Oct 16.

51.   Echtay KS, Esteves TC, Pakay JL, Jekabsons MB, Lambert AJ, Portero-Otin M, et al. A signalling role for 4-hydroxy-2-nonenal in regulation of mitochondrial uncoupling. EMBO J. 2003 Aug 15;22(16):4103-10.

52.   Uchida K, Shiraishi M, Naito Y, Torii Y, Nakamura Y, Osawa T. Activation of stress signaling pathways by the end product of lipid peroxidation. 4-hydroxy-2-nonenal is a potential inducer of intracellular peroxide production. J Biol Chem. 1999 Jan 22;274(4):2234-42.

53.   Lee S, Shin HS, Shireman PK, Vasilaki A, Van Remmen H, Csete ME. Glutathione-peroxidase-1 null muscle progenitor cells are globally defective. Free Radic Biol Med. 2006 Oct 1;41(7):1174-84.

54.   Kadenbach B. Intrinsic and extrinsic uncoupling of oxidative phosphorylation. Biochim Biophys Acta. 2003 Jun 5;1604(2):77-94.

55.   Smith RG, Henry YK, Mattson MP, Appel SH. Presence of 4-hydroxynonenal in cerebrospinal fluid of patients with sporadic amyotrophic lateral sclerosis. Ann Neurol. 1998 Oct;44(4):696-9.

56.   Clapham JC, Arch JR, Chapman H, Haynes A, Lister C, Moore GB, et al. Mice overexpressing human uncoupling protein-3 in skeletal muscle are hyperphagic and lean. Nature. 2000 Jul 27;406(6794):415-8.

57.   Ramsden DB, Ho PW, Ho JW, Liu HF, So DH, Tse HM, et al. Human neuronal uncoupling proteins 4 and 5 (UCP4 and UCP5): structural properties, regulation, and physiological role in protection against oxidative stress and mitochondrial dysfunction. Brain Behav. 2012 Jul;2(4):468-78.

58.   Hoffmann M. Vicious Circle of Metaboreflex Dysregulation in Amyotrophic Lateral Sclerosis. AASCIT Communications. 2014;1(2).

59.   Peters A, Schweiger U, Pellerin L, Hubold C, Oltmanns KM, Conrad M, et al. The selfish brain: competition for energy resources. Neurosci Biobehav Rev. 2004 Apr;28(2):143-80.

60.   Baek WS, Desai NP. ALS: pitfalls in the diagnosis. Pract Neurol. 2007 Apr;7(2):74-81.

61.   Lanni A, Moreno M, Lombardi A, Goglia F. Thyroid hormone and uncoupling proteins. FEBS Lett. 2003 May 22;543(1-3):5-10.

62.   Bacurau AV, Jardim MA, Ferreira JC, Bechara LR, Bueno CR, Jr., Alba-Loureiro TC, et al. Sympathetic hyperactivity differentially affects skeletal muscle mass in developing heart failure: role of exercise training. J Appl Physiol. 2009 May;106(5):1631-40.

63.   Murray AJ, Cole MA, Lygate CA, Carr CA, Stuckey DJ, Little SE, et al. Increased mitochondrial uncoupling proteins, respiratory uncoupling and decreased efficiency in the chronically infarcted rat heart. J Mol Cell Cardiol. 2008 Apr;44(4):694-700.

64.   Hoffmann M. Enhanced uncoupling of the mitochondrial respiratory chain as a potential source for amyotrophic lateral sclerosis. Front Neurol. 2013;4:86.

65.   Furby A, Beauvais K, Kolev I, Rivain JG, Sebille V. Rural environment and risk factors of amyotrophic lateral sclerosis: a case-control study. J Neurol. 2010 May;257(5):792-8.

66.   Abel EL. Football increases the risk for Lou Gehrig's disease, amyotrophic lateral sclerosis. Percept Mot Skills. 2007 Jun;104(3 Pt 2):1251-4.

67.   Wicks P, Ganesalingham J, Collin C, Prevett M, Leigh NP, Al-Chalabi A. Three soccer playing friends with simultaneous amyotrophic lateral sclerosis. Amyotroph Lateral Scler. 2007 Jun;8(3):177-9.

68.   Kamel F, Umbach DM, Munsat TL, Shefner JM, Hu H, Sandler DP. Lead exposure and amyotrophic lateral sclerosis. Epidemiology. 2002 May;13(3):311-9.

69.   Chio A, Calvo A, Dossena M, Ghiglione P, Mutani R, Mora G. ALS in Italian professional soccer players: the risk is still present and could be soccer-specific. Amyotroph Lateral Scler. 2009 Aug;10(4):205-9.

70.   Zhang CY, Parton LE, Ye CP, Krauss S, Shen R, Lin CT, et al. Genipin inhibits UCP2-mediated proton leak and acutely reverses obesity- and high glucose-induced beta cell dysfunction in isolated pancreatic islets. Cell Metab. 2006 Jun;3(6):417-27.

71.   Chen Y, Zhang H, Li YX, Cai L, Huang J, Zhao C, et al. Crocin and geniposide profiles and radical scavenging activity of gardenia fruits (Gardenia jasminoides Ellis) from different cultivars and at the various stages of maturation. Fitoterapia. 2010 Jun;81(4):269-73.

72.   Luo JZ, Luo L. American ginseng stimulates insulin production and prevents apoptosis through regulation of uncoupling protein-2 in cultured beta cells. Evid Based Complement Alternat Med. 2006 Sep;3(3):365-72.

73.   Ryu Y-J, Lee K-H, Kwon K-R, Lee Y-H, An J-C, Sun S-H, et al. Mountain Ginseng Pharmacopuncture Treatment on Three

Amyotrophic Lateral Sclerosis Patients. Journal of Pharmacopuncture. 2010;13(4):119-28.

74.   Johansen C, Olsen JH. Mortality from amyotrophic lateral sclerosis, other chronic disorders, and electric shocks among utility workers. Am J Epidemiol. 1998 Aug 15;148(4):362-8.

75.   Atherton PJ, Babraj J, Smith K, Singh J, Rennie MJ, Wackerhage H. Selective activation of AMPK-PGC-1alpha or PKB-TSC2-mTOR signaling can explain specific adaptive responses to endurance or resistance training-like electrical muscle stimulation. FASEB J. 2005 May;19(7):786-8.

76.   Beghi E, Pupillo E, Messina P, Giussani G, Chio A, Zoccolella S, et al. Coffee and amyotrophic lateral sclerosis: a possible preventive role. Am J Epidemiol. 2011 Nov 1;174(9):1002-8.

77.   Qureshi M, Shui A, Dibernardo AB, Brown RH, Jr., Schoenfeld DA, Cudkowicz ME. Medications and laboratory parameters as prognostic factors in amyotrophic lateral sclerosis. Amyotroph Lateral Scler. 2008 Dec;9(6):369-74.